The Guide of Raising Backyard Chickens

How To Do Breed Selection, Feeding, Care And Collecting Eggs For Beginners

Sally R. Ball

Table of Contents

Introduction

Chapter 1: Check the Laws in Your Area

Heritage Breeds

    Dark Brahma

    Ancona

    Araucana

Egg-Laying Breeds

    Leghorns

    Golden Comet

Dual-Purpose Breeds

    Rhode Island Red

    Sussex

    Australorps

Meat Breeds

    The Cornish Cross

The Guide Of Raising Backyard Chickens

Jersey Giants

Chapter 2: Getting Your Chicks for the First Time

How Many Chickens Should I Get?
Things to Look for When Buying Your Chicks

Chapter 3: Preparing the Coop
Chapter 4: Preparing for Chicks

Feed

Forms of Feed

When Can I Bring Them Outside for the First Time?
Pastured vs. Non-Pastured
Emergency Feed
Make or Buy Your Feed
Easy Routines

Chapter 5: Common Problems

Molting
Stopped Egg-Laying
Broodiness

Bullying

Predators

One May Be a Rooster!

Pasty Butt

Conclusion

The Guide Of Raising Backyard Chickens

Bluesource And Friends

This book is brought to you by Bluesource And Friends, a happy book publishing company.

Our motto is **"Happiness Within Pages"**

We promise to deliver amazing value to readers with our books.

We also appreciate honest book reviews from our readers.

Connect with us on our Facebook page www.facebook.com/bluesourceandfriends and stay tuned to our latest book promotions and free giveaways.

Don't forget to claim your FREE books!

Brain Teasers:

https://tinyurl.com/karenbrainteasers

Harry Potter Trivia:

https://tinyurl.com/wizardworldtrivia

Sherlock Puzzle Book (Volume 2)

https://tinyurl.com/Sherlockpuzzlebook2

Also check out our best seller book

https://tinyurl.com/lateralthinkingpuzzles

The Guide Of Raising Backyard Chickens

Description

Have you ever thought about raising your own backyard chickens? You might be surprised to find out that it's easier than you might think! Chickens can be a great addition to any household and are great fun for the whole family. They can provide copious amounts of eggs and meat.

This book will guide you through your journey of picking out your desired breed—there are hundreds! We will talk about a few great options depending on your wants and needs. Do you want chickens that will give you lots of eggs, or do you prefer chickens for meat? Once you clear that hurdle, we will show you where to purchase your chicks and what to look for when buying them. Stay clear of any anti-social behavior! What do you do when you get your birds home for the first time? You will most likely need a brooder if you are dealing with babies—or perhaps you'd like to try hatching them yourself with an incubator. How do you do that? This book will show you. We'll even give you some options if rearing babies sounds too hard for your first time around. How do you raise them, and what kind of attention do they need? What do they eat? Do they need a rooster?

We bring you right through adolescence to adulthood. What do you need for a wonderful coop that your girls will love? What is going to make your chickens the happiest? What is going to work best with you and your space? Do you have a big giant backyard with a fence, or will your ladies be more confined to the coop? We'll talk it through. We go through troubleshooting your flock to all the questions in between. Chickens can be fairly low maintenance and can provide a plentiful amount of benefits from healthy eggs and meat to land maintenance. For a complete guide to raising backyard chickens in almost any environment, look no further! Happy chicken rearing!

Introduction

Chickens are a type of domesticated fowl that originated from the red jungle fowl. They are extremely common and are widely used around the world. In 2011, there was an estimated total of 19 billion birds worldwide. With that number, chickens hold the largest population of any bird or domesticated fowl in the entire world. Many people are beginning to raise chickens in their backyards for both eggs and meat. They make great land keepers and offer many benefits. There are some things to know, however, before going into this adventure. Chickens and other fowl make a great addition to any household and provide eggs and meat as well as love and friendship.

Before you get your chicks, you need to ask yourself some questions. This book will help guide you through the exciting process of starting your backyard

The Guide Of Raising Backyard Chickens

chicken adventure. You will need to know the difference in breeds and be able to pinpoint your reason for keeping chickens. This book will bring you through all your chicken-rearing options—from hatching or buying day olds, to raising babies into egg-laying adults. Read this book if you're ready for a backyard adventure!

Chapter 1: Check the Laws in Your Area

Chickens shouldn't be a problem in rural areas, but if you are in the suburbs or urban area, you will want first to make sure that you are legally able to keep them with you. You will want to check city and state laws as well as any homeowners' association ordinances. There are many places that ban roosters because of noise issues as well as some that have a requirement for the number of chickens you can have. There are, indeed, places that impose this, so make sure that you clear this from a legal standpoint before you spend money or do any other research. It would be a shame to go through all this rewarding work only to have your chickens taken away in handcuffs. Just kidding. Do your research!

The Guide Of Raising Backyard Chickens

Congratulations on your decision to raise chickens in your backyard! That's great! You are on your way to a life of eggs, meat, and fun. Before we get started, there are some things to think about before your journey, which we will review in the next few paragraphs. To ensure a great life for your new backyard companions, you first want to strongly consider your reasons for getting them and a few logistical questions:

- Why do you want to raise chickens—eggs, meat, or pleasure?
- Where will you put the chickens?
- Do you have enough time?
- Are you willing to get "down and dirty" cleaning out their coop?
- Who will take care of them in long periods of your absence?
- Are you allowed to have chickens? If so, how many?

The Guide Of Raising Backyard Chickens

Maybe you have already thought of many of the answers to these questions, but do review and think about them nonetheless. Chickens can be a great lifestyle addition but do require a lot of time and attention that many people overlook. In many cases, chickens require just as much time and attention as any pet. Nobody wants their birds to suffer, so please take the time to make a decision thoughtfully.

Once you have decided that the chicken lifestyle is for you, then it's time to do a little research. Taking your time to research will ensure that you have the best experience and that your birds are as happy as can be.

Chickens have been a kitchen staple in American kitchens for hundreds of years. We wanted a hearty bird that could live long to produce eggs as well as be used for meat. You may think that there is just a "chicken," but you'd be wrong. There are breeds for different needs, and all breeds are not created equal. In today's world of industrial farming, chickens are not bred with sustainability in mind. Meat birds are injected with growth hormones to grow as quickly as possible. Years ago, it would take three times the amount of time to get half the amount of meat. Call me crazy, but I wouldn't want any of those growth hormones near my plate. Similarly, laying chickens are bred to lay as many eggs as possible, often losing flavor and most of the nutrients that come with wanting to eat eggs in the first place. Modern agriculture threatens chicken breed diversity since these birds are often hybrids and selected only for their ability to grow rapidly. Factory-farmed chickens account for over 90% of the chickens in America.

There are too many breeds of chicken to count. The number is estimated in the hundreds. There are birds that have been bred for specific reasons such as higher-quality meat, enhanced egg-laying, feathers for stuffing, and even fighting! While there may be too many breeds of chicken to count, they all fall into one of four categories. Let's go over a few in each of the categories.

Heritage Breeds

First up are heritage breeds. Heritage breeds are bred from lines that existed before the mid-20th century. The Livestock Conservancy, which is an American based organization to protect livestock states that a Heritage chicken is defined by being a naturally breeding chicken that grows slowly and can live a long and productive outdoor life. The American Poultry Association (APA) keeps a close watch on chicken breeding and states that a heritage breed is appropriate only if it is hatched from a heritage chicken that has been sired by an APA standard-bred chicken. Considering all of the aforementioned factory farming, we can say that it's easy to see why a heritage breed would be a great choice. Get a healthy and hearty bird that has stood the test of time and help resurrect some breeds from the brink of extinction. Some great examples of heritage breeds are:

Dark Brahma

The Dark Brahma is one of the largest of heritage chickens and is commonly referred to as "King of All Poultry." Their plumage is light and delicate with feathers on their feet! This breed was developed in Asia and first seen in America in the 1800s. They lay large brown eggs primarily in the months between October and May. The perfect supplement to any winter diet. However, their egg count is low with about three eggs per week per bird so choose your bird count accordingly. Because of their size, these birds also produce great meat. Their size also makes them the top of the pecking order in almost any flock but can also lead to some softer shelled eggs being accidentally squished. These birds are fairly laid back and don't mind confinement. The feathers on their feet can cause issues in cold, wet weather where mud can freeze and in some severe cases lead to frostbite. Cold and dry climates, however, work well for them because of their thicker feathering and a small comb.

Ancona

The Ancona came to America in 1888. Originally from Italy, they have a black and iridescent green feathering with white speckling. Their coat makes them great at hiding from predators, which works well with the fact that they are great foragers. The Ancona is particularly well-suited for farm life because of this. These birds are great for free range raising as they hate to be cooped up. Be sure you have enough space before deciding on this breed. Interestingly enough, these birds love to fly and may end up roosting elsewhere other than their coop. Keep an eye out for stray eggs, too! These birds are fairly rare which makes them a great option if you are passionate about saving heritage breeds from extinction. They lay medium white eggs and are hearty enough for cold weather while also being suitable for hot weather. Do note that this breed can be susceptible to frostbite.

Araucana

This breed is unusual, intelligent, weird and beautiful. The Araucana breed is originally from Chile but was bred further after coming to America. They lay a light blue or green egg and are often referred to as "Easter Eggers" even though that is a relative term to describe any breed that lays a light colored egg. These gorgeous colored eggs are one of the reasons people love these birds. These chickens are tufted rather than having traditional plumage which is very rare. The tufts almost look like moustaches made of feathers growing out of their necks. While some people love this trait, it does mean they are not great show birds as judges tend to not like this feature. This trait is actually a dominant and lethal gene. Then again, some people prefer this breed aesthetically. Their color is extremely varied. They are adapted to both hot and cold climates and are not susceptible to frostbite.

Egg-Laying Breeds

We then have egg-laying breeds which have been bred to have larger capacities for egg production, but this comes with a shorter production lifespan. Some great egg-laying hens are:

Leghorns

Originally named Italians, later being renamed Leghorns. This breed's heritage line originated in Tuscany, but the exact origin of what we, today, call the Leghorn, is unknown. It was brought to the states in the 1800s and is one of the most prolific breeds in modern industrial egg farming. While most people think of the Leghorn as being full white, with feathering and a red comb, they actually come in a variety of colors! Regardless, the white feathering these birds commonly have made them one of the most iconic looking breeds in America. The Leghorn is very intelligent and has proven to be highly self-sufficient and will be able to find a large majority of its food if given the opportunity to free-range. Because they love to range, they may also prefer to roost in trees. They are a high energy bird, so the more space, the better. They are known for becoming noisy if bored and cooped up for too long. They will lay around 250 to 300+ eggs a year that will be medium in size and white in color. This breed also has a bit of a longer egg-laying lifespan which is great for you! They make great beginner chickens but are not easy to train, so stay away from this breed if you are looking to tame your animals.

Golden Comet

The Golden Comet is a cross between a New Hampshire rooster and a White Rock hen and was bred specifically for egg production in the commercial-industrial sector but has since found its way to backyard farms all over the world. In fact, it is thought to be the most widely kept hybrid bird. An interesting thing to note is that this is actually not considered a breed, but a sex link chicken which is a bird that is sex-able upon hatching. This makes it almost fool-proof to tell the males and females apart, creating peace of mind for anyone buying them as chicks. No accidental rooster adoptions here! Their specific hybrid gives them a great combination of easy temperament while being both adaptable to hot and cold climates. This also means that they lay eggs earlier and give out large to extra-large eggs—as many as 330 per year. That's almost an egg a day! However, with this increased production comes a shorter lifespan. They are smaller—with the females weighing around 4 pounds, which then makes them great if you have kids around. While being a great size for backyards, these birds also have a great temperament and love human attention. They are resilient and can handle a wide range of climates. The name 'golden' comes from their cinnamon sugar colored coat with some possible white flecks.

Dual-Purpose Breeds

Up next we have dual-purpose breeds which are said to be the best of both worlds. These breeds do have a high egg-laying capacity, and they have an ability to grow large enough for them to be used for meat once they are older.

Rhode Island Red

The Rhode Island Red chicken breed is said to have been bred by a sailor after he bought a Malay rooster from a friend. He brought the rooster home to mate with his hens and then bred those babies. After a lot of cross-breeding and guessing, the Rhode Island Red was born. It was named state bird of Rhode Island in the 1950s. Unlike most breeds, Rhode Island Red chickens originated in America and are known as 'dual purpose' because they can provide both eggs and meat. They are often named one of the most successful breeds globally, as well as being an overall, extremely healthy breed. They have great personalities and love human interaction. They are brown and black contrary to their name. They are a popular backyard chicken because of their prolific egg-laying and their toughness. They will lay around 250 medium brown eggs a year. Their temperament ranges from very friendly to a little pushy and raucous with some noise mixed in, but they are considered to be low maintenance making them a great option for first-time chicken rearers.

Sussex

The Sussex breed originated from Sussex county in England and is considered one of the oldest English breeds. This graceful bird with great temperament and comes in eight color variations including silver, speckled, buff and brown. However, these exotic colors are becoming rarer with white being the most dominant color, currently. The Sussex breed is capable of laying 250 eggs per year while also being a great meat bird or 'broiler.' Eggs will vary from brown to cream, and the meat will be hearty. They have great temperament and are excellent for free ranging. This breed will eat right out of your hand! They are great 'beginner' birds due to their low maintenance nature. They survive well in a wide range of climates and do not have any serious health issues. This bird is great for families with kids and does well in a backyard situation.

Australorps

The Australorp is an Australian breed, originating from the Orpington breed. Commonly found with a soft black coat with showings of green and purple that twinkle in the sunlight along with their stark red gullets. They have been known to lay upwards of 300 eggs per year. They are also known for their friendly and docile temperament and seem particularly suited for backyard life as they are great with confinement, making them a superstar for backyard chicken breeders. They are great in cold climates but don't do as well in hotter weather.

Meat Breeds

Lastly, there are meat breeds which you can probably guess from the name are bred for their meat. They grow at an almost alarming rate putting on weight quickly and are ready for slaughter as early as nine weeks.

The Cornish Cross

This breed can reach twelve pounds in as little as six weeks but will be ready for harvest in as little as four weeks, making them the best meat bird available.

Though they grow rapidly, they maintain a great feed to weight ratio meaning making them a great investment. They grow and live well in most climates and are also great in confinement, but also make great pasture birds. They eat a lot, but grow fast and produce plenty of white meat. They taste better than most dual chicken breeds and are the top choice for many large farms as well as smaller backyard operations. These birds have a gentle nature and will serve as a friendly pet until it's time to process their meat. The best way to ensure these hens grow to their full potential is through the feeds you give them, so do some research on specific feed types as well as how and when, if this is the breed you end up choosing.

Jersey Giants

Originally bred in New Jersey to fill a hole in the market, the sheer size of these birds makes an impression. It is a mix of Black Java, Black Langshan and dark Brahmas and may contain some other, unknown breeds. Today, this breed is considered endangered and is rare to find in the states.

This bird was initially bred in the states to potentially replace the turkey, making it the biggest purebred breed in the states and potentially the world. Though it did not take over Turkey's place on our dinner tables, the breed was able to stake its own claim on the chicken world. These birds can reach up to thirteen pounds, but grow much slower than some other meat breeds, taking as much as twenty-one weeks to reach harvest. This makes them not suitable for commercial use, but highly favorable for backyard use while they are also calm and docile in nature.

Research is key when choosing your chicken breed. We've only covered a handful, and there are many other wonderful breeds. Make sure you know your needs and find a chicken breed to match them. Nobody wants a chicken putting on weight and ready

The Guide Of Raising Backyard Chickens

for slaughter after just nine weeks if they are looking for a plethora of eggs. For the most part, chicken breeds will mix and raise well together, so selecting multiple breeds is definitely an option.

Chapter 2: Getting Your Chicks for the First Time

Now that you have decided on what breeds of chicken that you want, it's time to purchase, and it can be hard to know where to start. You have a few different options when first getting your chicks, which we will review below—but for someone just starting out, there really is only one or two sensible options. You can hatch birds yourself and get babies, or you can get adults. In the end, it's about what you feel suits you the best, so let's take a look!

Hatching eggs would be the buying of fertilized eggs and using an incubator. Incubating eggs is fairly straightforward, but it is not recommended if you are new to chickens. There is a process, and although it's not difficult, you really need to have your pulse on

The Guide Of Raising Backyard Chickens

how to hatch using an incubator. If you really want to try your hand at it, then here are a few tips.

Interestingly enough, modern-day hens have become less attentive to their eggs—leaving a lot of farmers with trust issues when it comes to proper incubation and leading them to take it upon themselves. Incubators range from $50 up to the thousands. If you really want to invest, the higher-end incubators are super hands-off. In the eggs go and pop out baby chicks a few weeks later. If you aren't ready to shell out that kind of cash, then there are DIY options, but they require a ton of work. Regardless of where you fall on the incubator pricing scale, there are a few basic things that they all require.

Temperature needs to be kept at exactly 99.5 degrees at all times. Just one-degree difference can kill an egg. The humidity needs to be around 50% for about the first eighteen days and higher around 75% for the final days of incubation. Ventilation is also key. Egg shells are actually porous! Oxygen enters, and carbon dioxide exists—allowing the fetus chicks to breathe. Incubators need to have holes or vents to allow fresh air to reach the eggs.

A homemade incubator should involve some sort of insulated box like a Styrofoam cooler. A dimmable light bulb or heating pad will make a good heat source. You will need a pan of water and a sponge to create humidity. It's important to note that cheaper incubators will not consist of much more than this and can be a waste of money as they do not automate the temperature and humidity like higher-end models. You will want to invest in a good quality thermometer and hygrometer which measures humidity. I will stress good quality here as lower priced items will not be as accurate as needed. You can purchase a combination of the two with an external LED display. This will allow you to check the stats without disturbing the delicate environment. You will also want to purchase an automatic egg turner. This will save you time and take the guesswork out of egg turning. The finely tuned environment inside of the egg is kept just so by the constant rotation of the egg so don't skip this step. The incubator should be placed in a location with little to no heat fluctuation, like a basement. Avoid sunny areas and things like heat vents.

Unless you already have a flock with a rooster to fertilize eggs, you will need to find fertilized eggs from a local farm. It may sound silly, but the closer in proximity the farm is to the incubator the better it is for the eggs as the movement, and temperature fluctuations of travel can be detrimental even if for a short period of time. The less time, the better. Do not mail order your eggs.

Make sure to choose well-formed and full-size eggs that are clean, but do not clean them yourself. Doing so can disrupt the natural coat on the egg that is vital to the chick's success. Wash your hands before handling them and be as gentle as possible as any sudden movements can harm the embryo.

Once you have your fertilized eggs, it's time to incubate. You will want to have taken heat and humidity measurements from the incubator over a 24-hour period before placing the eggs into it, making whatever necessary adjustments to create the optimal environment. You can use less or more sponge surface depending on humidity needs. Adjust the lamp in small increments until 99.5 degrees is reached. Make sure to do this before picking up your eggs.

It will take roughly 21 days for hatching to occur once incubation begins. When you have reached your optimal incubator environment, it's time to introduce the eggs. You will want to keep an extremely close eye on temperature and humidity throughout the process and adjust accordingly. At day 18, add more water to

The Guide Of Raising Backyard Chickens

boost the humidity level. At this point, the eggs no longer need to be turned.

In the final days before hatching the eggs can be observed moving around on their own as the chick inside becomes ready to hatch. Eventually, it will peck a hole in the shell so that it can begin to breathe. Do not worry if the chicks then don't move. It can take up to twelve hours for their lungs to acclimate before they continue to peck their way out. Do not touch the eggs or attempt to help them hatch as they are very fragile and it's quite easy to cause injury. Once the chick has broken free, you will want to let it dry off in the warmth of the incubator before moving it to the brooder.

If this process seems too expensive or labor-intensive, but you want to enjoy the delight that comes with having baby chicks around, then buying day-old chicks is for you. This option is easier than incubating and buying chicks is fairly cheap. This option is highly recommended for first-time chick owners.

You will first want to find a local farm or garden store that has the desired breed and coordinate with them on hatching schedules. Take advantage of store staff as they can answer most questions you might have. It's also a convenient one-stop-shop as most of these stores or farm stands will have everything you need to get started. An advantage to buying from the store is the chicks will tend to be a little older as they won't sell all of them at once. Older chicks tend to be healthier, more resilient and require a little less care.

You also have the option of ordering chicks online which is less expensive. It may seem crazy, but there are dozens of farms all around the country that ship newborns directly to your doorstep. This is a great option if you are looking for a specific breed. They do usually require a minimum of around 25 or 50, so that is something to keep in mind.

The Guide Of Raising Backyard Chickens

Another buying option is to get pullets. A pullet is a grown to adulthood bird that is just about to start laying eggs. They will be considerably more expensive than baby chicks and also eat more. The upside is that you have not had to waste time, money, and energy to raise chicks. You can get right to the egg-laying! This is definitely something to think about as most people really love the connection that comes with having them as babies.

With pullets, you eliminate the cost of chick rearing but immediately spend more on food and the bird itself. You can weigh the pros and cons for yourself and make a decision based on what's best for you.

However, adult hens are another option—it can be hard to come by, as most breeders move out older birds due to higher feeding costs. Hence, if you are looking for ample amounts of eggs, you should also steer clear as chickens are at their egg-laying peak for the first 1-2 years after their first egg. Adopting older hens from shelters is a great option for people looking to rescue animals.

How Many Chickens Should I Get?

The number of birds you order depends on your own personal needs. Are you using them for eggs? If so, what breed are you getting? Strong egg-laying breeds will produce 5-6 eggs a week. How many eggs does your family eat? Think about all of those things and then do some maths. Generally speaking, six healthy birds will average 4 eggs per day. Always err on the side of having a couple of extra chickens just to be safe. Having too many eggs is a good problem to have as you can most likely easily give them away.

If you are using the chickens for meat, then you will need to do the maths for that. Most likely you will need more than for eggs considering the time it takes to get to maturity, and you might be averaging one or two roast chickens a week. You will also want to keep in mind the lifecycles and plan accordingly.

Things to Look for When Buying Your Chicks

The birds should have clear, bright eyes. They should be interactive with you, the other chicks, and their surroundings. Their fluff should be clean and have good coloring. Things to avoid are birds that exhibit sleepiness, nasal and eye discharge, or any anti-social behaviour like sitting away from the flock. Avoid birds with any of these traits. Above all, use your judgment and look for healthy birds.

Chapter 3: Preparing the Coop

In layman terms, a coop is the chicken house. Chickens don't need much in terms of housing, but there are some necessities to keep in mind to ensure that your birds are safe and cared for.

Some basics include the shelter itself, of course. You can certainly Google some plans if you'd like to build your own—a place for your chickens to hide away from the more extreme weather elements. Make sure that it is water and weatherproof. You will also want to make sure there is enough space so that your chicks don't feel claustrophobic. When space is too tight, some chickens will start pecking one another, especially in colder weather. Ventilation is also crucial for temperature control. Just like your house, you want it to be cooler in summer months and warmer in the winter. For this to work, you need good airflow. Ventilation holes work well for this. Don't worry too

The Guide Of Raising Backyard Chickens

much about temperature, as chickens can survive in below freezing weather as long as you have the correct breeds. Make sure to keep attention on whether or not the coop is too hot. Any temperatures above 90 degrees can lead to health issues for your chickens. You can combat this issue by giving your coop more ventilation and ensuring a great cross breeze. You can also consider a misting fan if the issue is really persistent.

You will also need nesting boxes for your chickens to lay eggs. They are not actually essential for egg-laying. A chicken will lay eggs wherever they feel safe, but a nesting box makes it way more likely that the eggs can be found in them every time rather than scattered around the yard. The boxes must be quiet, safe, on the darker side, and private. These attributes help to make the chicken feel safe and in turn, give you more eggs. The boxes should be placed in a darker area of the coop that is low traffic. They can be anywhere from 18 inches to a few feet off of the ground, though not as high as the roosting bars. This will avoid confusion as to where they should be sleeping. Being off the ground ensures cleanliness and that they are away from predators. One box for every three birds is plenty good, and you can go as high as five hens per box, but shy away from anything higher than that as it can be considered inhumane. For a standard hen, each box should be a 12-inch cube. Larger birds, such as the Jersey Giant, will need the width to be around 14 inches in order to accommodate their larger size. You want the box to be snug to the bird to keep it clean and to discourage birds from rooming together. Some great options for nesting materials are pine shavings, straw, pine needles, sawdust, and leaves. Any and all of these can be used alone or combined. Also, the addition of lavender and lemon balm to the boxes will help the girls relax and deter pests. They are highly recommended! Don't worry if they all clamor for the same box. It's very common for there to be a favorite nesting box. The hens also need to be trained to lay eggs in the boxes. Usually putting a golf ball or fake egg into the nester BEFORE they start laying will give them the idea.

Chickens prefer to be high up off of the ground when they sleep. They are great sleepers and being off the ground guards against predators as well as pathogens, bacteria, and parasites. All of this means you need a good roost. A roost is a perch or beam for chickens to sleep on at night. For the most part, they will all sleep together because there is safety in numbers, but don't be alarmed if one or two shy away from the crowd. Chickens take their pecking order seriously and those higher in the pecking order will claim higher parts of the perch. This leaves those below more vulnerable. Some great makeshift bars include hearty branches, ladders, and planks. You'll want a minimum of 2 inches wide, preferably 4 inches. A 2'x4' with the thick part facing up works very well.

The Guide Of Raising Backyard Chickens

You want to avoid metal and plastic, and it will be hard to grip for the birds and metal can get very cold. Chickens poop while they sleep so make sure to place the bar in a convenient location for yourself to clean and also away from any food or water. You can place it anywhere more than a foot off the ground. If it's more than two feet, try to stagger a few, so it's easier for them to get up and down. Also, make sure to leave a fifteen-inch clearance from the ceiling, so they have more than enough headspace. One hen requires about eight inches of space. Do the math accordingly.

You will also want to consider security measures when putting your coop together as predators are around 24/7 and come in all shapes and sizes. Avoid chicken wire as it does not protect against predators coming in. Look for smaller wire around 1/2". Be sure to layer some of the same wire underneath both the coop and the run to protect against any animal that loves to dig. Be sure there is a secure roof, of course. This will also protect against the weather. Be sure to use quality locks and to check them nightly. You may also want to consider some lighting that is motion censored as it will deter predators right from the start. Lastly, if you think larger predators like bears may be an issue in your area, consider putting an electric fence around the coop for extra security.

Now that you have the coop all set up, you need to ensure that your hens have ample outside space. Depending on your own situation, this can be free range or a contained, fenced in space.

You'll need to decide if you are going to free range your chickens or keep them in a fenced area. There are pros and cons to each so let's take a look.

Free-range chickens tend to have a more varied diet and therefore better nutrients which leads to better eggs and meat. Free range can be a great option, but not everyone has space and capacity for it. There are some things you will want to consider when deciding.

Chickens will roam without a fence, so unless you are on a big farm, you will want a fence. Even on a farm, you will most likely still want a barrier as your chickens can be more susceptible to predators. You will also want to consider that there will be poop in your yard which is bad for bare feet, but great for fertilizing. Chickens will most likely dig one or two dust baths that will look like brown dirt circles on your grass. You will also want to make sure your garden is protected as chickens will not shy away from eating veggies.

Having chickens in a confined pen will definitely keep things cleaner and may be necessary for more urban outdoor areas. The chickens will still have access to some grub from the lawn, but will definitely have to be supplemented with feed. A chicken run is great if

The Guide Of Raising Backyard Chickens

you don't want them to have total lawn access, but of course, want to give them outdoor space.

Chapter 4: Preparing for Chicks

Okay—the day has come, and you are ready to welcome your new backyard friends into their new home. If you have decided to go with baby chicks, then the following will help you prepare for their arrival.

You will want to make sure that you have all of your supplies ready to go. Whether you ordered online or have gone to a farm store, you'll want to ensure a full set up before your new additions arrive.

You'll want to make sure that you have a brooding box, which can range from something like a cardboard box to something more sophisticated purchased online or at the store. It's simply a heated, enclosed area to house your new chicks while they begin to grow. If this is your first time, it may be wise to go with the cheapest option. You can always

The Guide Of Raising Backyard Chickens

upgrade later. Whatever you choose, make sure it's tall enough so they don't jump out and that there is enough room for the chicks, the water, and food. You also want to consider a cover if you think there might be predators. This includes household pets. To ensure safety, you can simply use chicken wire to create a cover that is well ventilated. You'll want to keep them in here for about 6-8 weeks until their feathers come in and they seem more confident in their surroundings. You'll know it's time when they are no longer the cute yellow fluff balls you first welcomed. At a minimum, a brooder should have heat (preferably non-flammable), food, water source, and bedding.

The easiest route for heat is a heat lamp, but beware that they can be considered fire hazards. You especially want to stay away from heat lamps if there is cardboard anywhere in your brooding box. A heating plate is a more expensive, but safer option.

The Guide Of Raising Backyard Chickens

You'll want to keep your chicks at about 100 degrees for the first week, reducing 5-10 degrees every week. Your chicks won't have feathers until about 8 weeks and therefore cannot regulate their body temperatures. Rather than keeping a thermometer, you can simply look at the chick's behavior. If they are pressed against the outskirts of the brood away from the lamp, they are too hot. If they are huddled together, it would be too cold—you want them to be scattered evenly throughout the brood. That's when you know the temperature is just right.

There are a lot of options when it comes to food. You can make your own, but for simplicity sake, you might want to start with starter feed from the store. The chicks will want to eat this for the first 8 weeks then you can mix it with grow feed for another 4-8 weeks. Add finisher feed 15-18 weeks, then layer feed at 18 weeks plus. Feed comes either medicated or not. The main reason is to defend against coccidiosis, a nasty disease we will talk about in the next chapter. Ask the person you purchased the chicks from if the chicks have been vaccinated. You can then make an informed decision when purchasing the feed. When you first get the chicks into the brooder, you will want to dip the beak of each chick into the food gently. They will be able to locate the food on their own after this.

Once the chicks turn into pullets, you will want to lower their protein intake. This will slow their growth, but ensure strong bones and proper body weight before the egg-laying begins. You will feed them this until they are fourteen weeks old and then move onto feed.

Feed

There are many different types of feed that you will feed to your birds throughout their lives. What kind will depend on the age of the flock and for what purpose you are raising them—meat or eggs?

You will start with the chick starter. You will feed them this type for the first six weeks while they remain infants. This is about 20% protein for egg layers—a little more for meat birds. You will have to decide if you want to be medicated or not. Most use medicated, but smaller farms and those who practice a more organic take on raising chickens may not.

We then have grower pullet. When chicks mature into pullets that will be egg layers their protein intake is reduced to slow growth and focus on building strong bones and proper adult weight for laying eggs. If the chick's protein levels continue and they grow too quickly, it can lead to complications.

At 14 weeks, you then switch to pullet developer/finisher. This will lower their protein even more right before laying. It is important to note that

The Guide Of Raising Backyard Chickens

some feed companies do not distinguish between these two different pullet feeds and sometimes combine both of them into one with a medium amount of protein between the two.

Layer rations are fed at around 22 weeks. This feed averages 17% protein but has added calcium and minerals to ensure proper eggshell strength. Please do not feed this to any chicken younger than 22 weeks as it can severely damage the kidneys of the bird due to high amounts of calcium and phosphorus.

Broiler rations are, you guessed it, for broiler chickens. This is high-protein feed to produce hearty meat. Birds can be reduced to 16% after 12 weeks. They can live on this until butchering. Some may want to keep them on a heavier protein. It's really up to you.

One thing to note is that pasture-raised chickens do require less feed. If you are looking for ways to save money on feed, this is a great option. It also creates a better diet for your birds. Pasture-raised birds get the pleasure of eating wildflowers and grasses as well as small insect and worms. This ups their nutrient intake and leads to better harvests.

Forms of Feed

Chicken food comes in three basic forms: crumbles, pellets, and mash. Crumbles are great, but they are sometimes hard to come by and often, pellets are the only form available. Mash is usually fed to baby chicks, but a lot of people love mixing it with warm water. It makes an oatmeal-like substance. Chickens love this! This mash quickly becomes moldy, however, so must be eaten right away and not left to sit around and harden.

Bear in mind that chicks are messy. They love playing with their food and throwing it around. Just like real babies! They poop in their feeders and make a mess of their bedding. Ask your farm stand or farmer what feeder they recommend when you pick up your chicks.

Water is, of course, an essential when it comes to any living creature. When you first get your chicks, you can gently put their beaks into the water, so they know where to find it, just as you did with the food. You will also want to make sure the water is not too hot or cold. Any feed store, as well as online outlets, will have cheap chick waterers. Try to avoid open bowls as this can lead to young chicks drowning. If you are in a pinch, you can put marbles in the bottom of the bowl for the first few weeks to prevent chick loss due to drowning. You will also want to add electrolyte supplements to the water for the first couple weeks to ensure proper hydration. In addition, you will need to check and change the water multiple times per day to keep the area clean. Your new friends can be messy, and you want to make sure there isn't food and bedding in the water.

A great and affordable bedding option is pine shavings. These help to soak up moisture and keep the chicks from slipping on the floor. You can also add paper towels to the base level of the floor to keep slippage at a minimum. You want to make sure the birds aren't slipping as this can lead to walking and leg development issues. Other options can be sand or animal training pads.

Hygiene is another important aspect of keeping a brooder. It will differ from person to person depending on what you're comfortable with. You definitely want to keep things clean, but don't necessarily need to sanitize. Keep in mind that, like humans, especially children, a little dirt is actually good for the immune system, and completely stripping bacteria away can actually be detrimental to the immune system. That being said, there a few rules of thumb to go by. The chicks will be pooping all over the brooder, and you will need to clean accordingly. The poop will be warm and wet which is a great place for bacteria to grow. Make sure to be cleaning this out as often as needed. Once the bedding is wet, it really must be changed. You will want to wash and or sanitize the feeder and waterer a few times a week. Use your discretion. Some batches of chicks will be messier than others! Trust your gut and what you feel is right for you and your chicks. One thing to keep in mind is to throw out any food from a feeder that has been pooped in. Even if you think it hasn't touched anything, you want to be safe. And for safekeeping, wash your hands before and after handling chicks.

Security is another issue that you want to make sure you have a handle on, or it could lead to devastating results. You will want your brooder to be away from any predators, and that includes house pets. With that in mind, you may want to consider avoiding highly trafficked areas as there can be a lot of dust kicked into the air by these fluff balls. A garage or barn can be a great location as long as they have secure entries and no rats are nearby. Larger predators may be obvious, but rats won't shy away from chomping into a chick. Beware!

Please be aware that your chicks will need constant attention until they reach roughly 12 weeks old.

When Can I Bring Them Outside for the First Time?

You will want to wait until your chicks are at least four weeks old before bringing them outside for the first time and only then if the weather outside is warmer to hot. Remember that they will still need to be kept warm. To be safe, you may want to wait until the chicks are feathered around eight to twelve weeks.

A dog crate works great for bringing chicks outside. Make sure to place them in some shade, so the food and water don't get too hot. Ideally, half shade and half sun so they can choose. You will also want to monitor their behavior to ensure they are comfortable. It will also give you an idea of how to handle bringing them outside on future outings. Of course, you will also want to ensure their outside cage is also predator proof.

Pastured vs. Non-Pastured

Now that you've successfully reared a brood, the hard part is mostly over. You have given your love and devotion to these birds for months now, and it is time to let them be self-sufficient (mostly). There are things to keep in mind when it comes to adult chicken basics.

Again, water is essential. An adult hen will drink about a cup of water a day. You can multiply that by how many birds you have, and that's how much water you should have at all times. Keep in mind that for larger flocks you might want to have a few different water sources spread throughout the living space. The easiest way to water is to buy a drinker.

Food is, of course, a key ingredient for any animal. Here is a quick guide to what you might want to feed your chickens. You should start with what birds eat in the pasture. This includes grasses like clover and buckwheat, weeds, and other vegetation. Chickens will also eat insects like earthworms and slugs. In addition, they will need some grit in their diet like sand and dirt. They keep this in their gizzards to help them grind up the aforementioned foraged foods.

You will want your chickens to get as much foraged and natural food as possible. When a hen's diet consists of large amounts of food from mother nature, you can truly see the difference in her eggs. The yolks have a deep orange color and thick, viscous

The Guide Of Raising Backyard Chickens

whites. The meat will also be denser and tender from pasture-raised chickens as well as have a higher omega-3 content. That being said, you will most likely need to supplement with feed as this is the guide to backyard chickens and most backyards, depending on where you live, don't have enough grass to provide proper feed for more than a couple chickens.

If you can't fully raise your chickens on pasture, you might want to consider having a fenced area outside of the coop (a run) where they can get exercise and hopefully grab a supplemental worm or two. They will be happier and healthier. Do keep in mind that if you do pasture your chickens that you will want to make sure they are safe from predators either with a protected area or with a guard dog.

Backyard chickens can eat scraps from the household, but you will want to avoid foods like beans, garlic, potatoes, onions, and citrus as they can be harmful

You can also consider some supplements for any commercial feed. Oyster shells are an unexpected but wonderful addition as they have tons of calcium. Cabbage and grit (sand or dirt) are other things to be introduced. Especially grit, as they need it to help digest vegetation. The more diversity in nutrients, the better. Do make sure to double check online if you are unsure about what human food is safe for them.

Emergency Feed

In an emergency, if you run out of feed, you can chop up hard boiled eggs and feed them to your chickens. It seems a little barbaric, but it works in a pinch. Chickens are also able to go a couple of days without feed and subside off of kitchen scraps for a little bit of time. The same doesn't go for water. Make sure they always have ample amounts of water.

The Guide Of Raising Backyard Chickens

Make or Buy Your Feed

It's important to point out that you have a variety of choices when it comes to your feeds. You can design, buy, and mix in many ways. You may wish to buy store-bought pellets and add in some of your own vegetation. You can grow your own seeds, grasses, and grains. Any store-bought feed will have varying directions as far as specific age to feed your chicks certain things. This will differ by brand. Be sure to check—do your research. When in doubt, you can ask your local feed store, and don't forget to keep an eye on nutrition content if you decide to make your own.

There are many different options when it comes to chicken feed. You can purchase feed at the store which is, of course, the easiest. You can design and mix your own feed with a combination of store-bought, kitchen scraps and even grow your own grains and seeds.

In addition to water, the other key thing a chicken does need is food.

Giving your chickens the correct food will keep them happy and turn them into an egg-laying machine. Give them the wrong food, and it can lead to all sorts of problems including bullying and weight loss.

Easy Routines

It's great when you can give lots of time and attention to your hens, but this is not always the case. Here are some essential guidelines for what needs to be done daily.

When you get up in the morning, you can let your coop open, either to the run or to pasture. Get those ladies outside! You will want to check their food and water levels. Give the coop a once over to make sure everything seems in good standing.

The Guide Of Raising Backyard Chickens

In the evening, when the sun sets you will want to bring your girls back inside and make sure all locks are secure. Grab whatever eggs may be inside and kiss them good night.

This is the very least you can do for your chickens, and there will most definitely be more work here and there. You will need to do weekly chores such as cleaning the coop and fixing the nesting beds.

Chapter 5: Common Problems

Raising chickens is fairly straightforward and easy. They can add great value to any household, but do come with things to think about. It's a fact of life that at least one of your chickens will most likely suffer. There are ways to circumvent issues that may seem more alarming than they actually are. Here is a list of some common chicken issues.

Moulting

Molting is a process that all chickens go through. It's when they lose old, worn-out feathers and replace them with new plumage and usually happens in the fall when they are preparing for winter. Aside from initial molts in their first year of life, chickens molt about once a year. The first molt actually happens quite early at about six to eight days when they replace their fluffy down with feathers. After two or three months, they replace their baby feathers with adult ones. All birds, including roosters, do this. The typical length of a molt is three months, but some birds can take up to two years to complete the process. The loss of feathers starts at the head and goes south down the body. Some chickens will lose all feathers at once, leaving them looking bare, and others will do it more gradually and just have some patchiness. The look can range from severe to not noticeable. Again, this takes about three months and is usually triggered by a decrease in sunlight hours. Cool! Chickens may also slow egg production at this time. You will want to make sure the health of your birds is top-notch during this process by increasing their protein. Seeds, nuts, peas, and soybeans are great snacks to help raise protein levels. Make sure to keep an eye on your chickens at this time as their behavior may be off. They tend to have decreased energy, but you want to monitor to ensure they aren't sick.

Any grown chicken that is losing feathers at other times of year should be looked at. Feather loss that is not molting can be due to stress, parasite infestation, and inadequate diet. If you suspect mites, you can use natural oils to deter and keep them away. Lavender, wormwood, mint, and lemon balm all help deter unsavory creatures from the coop. Vaseline is specifically recommended for scaly leg mites. You can spray need oil in the coop. Again, to get a solid diagnosis you will want to talk to a vet and get a treatment recommendation.

Some other signs of sickness are:

- A pale and limp comb (could be the cause of frostbite or worms)

    Try this: Chickens are fairly good at mustering through cold weather, but frostbite still occurs. You can try applying a warm cloth to warm the area slowly.

- Coughing, wheezing, or runny nose (could be respiratory disease)

    Try this: Ensure the coop is clean with as little dust as possible. A quick clean of the coop can clear up any or most of these symptoms. Also, make sure there is proper ventilation to make sure your birds are getting fresh, clean air. If symptoms persist, call a vet.

- Heavy breathing and holding wings away from the body (maybe heat stroke)

    Try this: Spray them with water to help with the heat. You can also try some ice cubes and frozen food. Make sure they have access to water and shade.

These are a few common health issues. It is always a great rule of thumb to call a vet when in doubt about the health of your birds. Getting a professional opinion will make sure the birds recover quickly and give you peace of mind.

Stopped Egg-Laying

It can be scary if your girls stop laying eggs. Are they sick or are the eggs hidden away somewhere? Some of the most common reasons are:

- Molting at 15–18 months will end egg-laying for a while.
- Chickens need about 15–16 hours of light a day, and if they don't get it, it may harm the egg-laying.
- Diet can be an issue if they are not receiving enough nutrients.
- Dehydration can also be an issue. Make sure, especially in hot weather, that your girls are getting enough water.

- The eggs could also be getting stolen by predators. Even humans have been known to steal eggs!
- A change in the pecking order may also cause stress and drama within the pecking order. This can throw off the hens.

Broodiness

A broody hen wants to hatch its own eggs. The behavior is described as constantly sitting in the nest, squawking, grumbling, and puffing her chest. Some ways you can get her to stop are: removal, closing down the nest, a cold water drip, by removing all materials or cut off access to the coop.

Bullying

Bullying does occur due to the subtleties of the pecking order. Each hen should know her place, but every flock has some trouble makers. If a hen goes out of turn, she may receive a peck from another to put her in her place. It shouldn't become too extreme, but you can quickly research some ideas if it does.

Predators

You will always have predators, even in urban areas. Make sure to have some sort of fence in place if you are allowing your girls to run free. This will keep them from wandering off. You may also want to consider a chicken/fowl watchdog. The key to security is to make sure the coop is locked down at night and that the chicks have security measures in place during the day. Make sure to secure underneath the coop as well to keep out any animals that are good at digging. You can revisit coop security from the earlier chapters.

One May Be a Rooster!

There is a 10% chance that you will receive a rooster (male) when you get your chicks. You will know for sure when they go through their second molt, which is when their ornamental feathers start to come in. A lot of urban areas have laws against roosters for noise reasons. If this becomes an issue, reach out to a local farm and see if they will take him in.

Pasty Butt

Pasty butt is a baby chick affliction. This is when poop builds up and blocks their rear end. It can be fatal if not treated but is easily taken care of. This only affects young chicks in the brooder. It's caused by inconsistent heat within their brooder. Using a radiant heater will usually eliminate this altogether. To fix this, take a warm damp cloth and wipe the chick where it's blocked a couple of times a day for a week. It should be cleared up by then.

Conclusion

There you have it—your backyard guide to raising chickens. Don't forget to do your research, make informed decisions, and use your instincts. All chicks are not created equal, and it may require a little tweaking here and there. Raising chicks can be very rewarding for the entire family, but it is not something to casually throw yourself into. You don't want to make this decision lightly, so take the time to consider your breed and what use you want from your chickens. Make sure that you will have the proper time to care for these new household companions. Consider space and time management. Make sure that your chicks have ample amounts of healthy food and water. Do your best to protect them with security measures to avoid any issues with predators. Don't forget to check your local laws before beginning. The best of luck in your backyard chicken adventures!

The Guide Of Raising Backyard Chickens

Sally R. Ball

The Guide Of Raising Backyard Chickens

Connect with us on our Facebook page www.facebook.com/bluesourceandfriends and stay tuned to our latest book promotions and free giveaways.

Manufactured by Amazon.ca
Bolton, ON